A Weigh To Lose

Tips For A Successful Weight Loss Journey

Kim McPherson

A Weigh To Lose

Thank you for purchasing this book. By purchasing this book you are not only getting information on weight loss, you are also supporting my dream to become an entrepreneur.

Sign up for our newsletter and get great recipes, plus weight loss and fitness tips by emailing us at aweightolose@gmail.com

Check it out on our website and our social media accounts:

Website: www.aweightolose.com

Facebook: www.facebook.com/aweightolose

Twitter: @aweightolose

Instagram: @aweightolose

www.ingramcontent.com/pod-product-compliance
Lightning Source LLC
Chambersburg PA
CBHW070107290526
45789CB00005B/1951

Table of Contents

My Journey

Since I started my business, I have always been told to share my personal journey. I have struggled with my weight since I was a pre-teen. I also began suffering from self-esteem issues at a young age. I learned very quickly how to beat myself up mentally, and those habits were embedded in my brain.

Portion control was non-existent, and I was always told to clean my plate. Growing up, I went through several rough patches and I learned very quickly to turn to food. Food became my comfort and my crutch. Also, I loved hanging out with friends. It was my escape for when things were bothering me. Hanging out with friends always involved food. No matter what we were doing we would always eat, and it was always fast food because we couldn't afford anything else.

All I cared about was if it tasted good. Growing up, I never thought about calories or nutritional content of my food. I wasn't educated on the benefits of nutritious food and nor did I care. I was more concerned about escapism; getting away from my problems through distractions and food.

I learned these habits at a young age and continued with these habits through adulthood. Throughout my life, I have done diets and weight loss programs. I would lose weight but always fall off the wagon and end up gaining more weight. I've never successfully finished a diet. As I got older more stresses entered my life along with more happiness. Getting married to the love of my life changed so many things for me. I was also blessed to have a stepdaughter.

I always wanted to do everything I could to take care of them and give them the best life possible. Eight years ago, I decided to go back to school. Professionally this was a blessing and one of the smartest decisions I have made. Personally, it was detrimental to my health. I worked full-time and went to school at night. Fast food became a convenience.

I would eat late at night and my stress level was overwhelming. I was also getting minimal sleep, which only created a more toxic mix to my life. I was miserable and hated myself so much I avoided mirrors and constantly berated myself. This made things worse, causing me to turn to food for comfort, and I became a food addict.

I literally fantasized about food. I remember looking up food on Pinterest or watching cooking shows hoping it would curb my cravings. I thought it would stop me from eating; instead it made me want food even more.

Having the love to cook was also harmful to my waistline. My focal point for cooking was making food taste the absolute best it could. The more calories the better was my motto. I never used substitutes to reduce calories because I thought it would detract from the pleasure of the food I was preparing. I also got enjoyment from others eating the food I cooked. It gave me such pleasure to receive compliments on my cooking. The reason for this was because it made me feel good. It would temporarily boost my self-esteem.

Going back to school and my obsession with food caused my weight to skyrocket. I thought once I finished school that I would be able to get my weight under control. However, I was wrong. I got a new job right out of college and the job was very demanding. I became so career-focused, I didn't care about my personal health. I continued the same habits as I always did and continued to gain weight.

Two years ago, I decided as always to set a New Year's resolution. I did this every year, and the goal was always the same - to lose weight. My husband decided to join me on this journey since over the years he had gained weight as well. My choices and self-destructive behavior towards food had also affected him.

In the beginning, we did well. I fell off the wagon but would quickly climb back on. My husband did much better than I did. His resolve was strong and he had a better focus on his plan. Throughout this journey, I continued to struggle but kept going.

I struggled with my workouts. Embarrassment plagued me every time I went to the gym. People even laughed at me and there were many nights I went home crying. However, I was determined to not give up, and I learned to keep my focus entirely on my workout while blocking out the negativity that surrounded me at the gym.

Eight months into this journey I got frustrated. I was fed up and wanted to quit. I knew that wasn't a solution, but I was so desperate to lose weight I didn't know what to do. I decided that I should consider drastic measures. I began considering weight loss surgery.

I didn't take this decision lightly. I did some research and talked about it with my husband. Once my mind was made up, I found a doctor and attended his seminar. I also discussed my plans with his client coordinator. I even spoke to my insurance and the hospital where the surgery would be held. I wanted to make sure I covered all my bases.

I was concerned about paying for the surgery and originally opted against it because of the cost, but out of desperation, I decided the benefit outweighed the cost.

I was all set to move forward. All I needed to do was schedule the surgery. I was trying to find the perfect time to schedule surgery so that it wasn't too hard for my co-workers as well as my husband and step daughter. While I was contemplating this, that persistent little voice in my hand asked me if I was really to the point that surgery was my only option. I knew that I was going to schedule my surgery several months out. I decided that it wouldn't hurt to try one more time before I scheduled my surgery.

Since I was going to give traditional weight loss one last shot, needed to do something different. I wanted to try a completely different approach. The first thing I did was to take some of the diets I had done in the past and analyze them. I reviewed what the diet was about, how it worked, and why it failed. I chose some healthy diets, quick fix diets, and a few fad diets.

As I was going through them, I saw a pattern. All the diets were different in their own way. However, they had something in common—failure. The reason the diets failed were not the fault of the diet. I was the reason the diet failed.

I couldn't stay focused on my goals. I was the reason I wouldn't stick to the program. Once I realized that I was the problem and not the diet, everything clicked. I shifted my focus to mental motivation, and it all fell into place.

I created my own meal plan and designed my own workout plan. To this day I continue to use the program that I developed on my own. Thanks to my hard work I have managed to lose over 110 pounds in the past two years.

I became so passionate about my journey that I wanted to help others. I was going through some changes at work and realized it was time to venture out on my own and become an entrepreneur. I chose to create a business around my journey and take what I have learned and experienced and help others.

Losing weight is a journey. It is important to make this your own journey. Your journey could be a short or long. In either case your weight loss journey will always be a part of your life.

Losing weight is hard. It is a constant battle many of us face every day. A lot of us have been there. We have tried numerous diets only to fail miserably. The truth is there are diets that work. Yes, you just read that. Not all diets work but there are healthy balanced diets that can deliver the results.

The diet is not the problem. The problem is ourselves. We become so focused on the diet and exercise plan that we fail to focus on the most important aspect and that is mental motivation. Without it we don't eat right nor do we exercise. The book will provide tips on meal plans, exercise plans, and how to stay motivated while participating in any weight loss program. Always remember, you should consult your primary physician before starting any weight loss or fitness program.

Most weight loss program consist mainly of two components: meal plans and exercise. I don't believe there are any special pills, potions, or products to help you lose weight and keep it off. I believe in the tried and true way. I also believe this is the best way to reach long-term success with our weight loss journey. Unfortunately, you will have to do this the hard way which is the old-fashioned way —diet and exercise. There is hope and you can do this.

A great weight loss program consists of three things; meal plan, exercise plan, and mental motivation. Each of these will be discussed in detail.

Meal Plan Tips

The first item we will discuss is your meal plan. When selecting a meal plan make sure it is one that is feasible for you to do. You want a meal plan that fits your lifestyle. Before you choose any meal plan, review it, and make sure it is a plan you can follow. It has to be flexible to fit your needs. Going too restrictive can be detrimental to your success.

Most meal plans involve meal preparation. Meal prep is a great way to stay on your meal plan. Preparing foods ahead of time for your week will save time and money. Here are some tips when doing meal prep.

Set time aside each week for meal prep. Most people prefer to do this on the weekend.

Invest in meal prep containers. These are great as they store and stack well. They are also affordable. Amazon has several types of affordable containers.

You can also slowly try incorporating healthier foods into your family's diet.

If meal prep isn't your thing, there are alternatives. Have someone else prep your meals or try a meal delivery service. You can also check out your local grocery store. T.V. dinners have come a long way. There are some healthy frozen meals you can purchase at affordable prices. Next time you are in your local grocery store, check out the frozen food section and see what you can find.

Log your meals. Using a free app to keep track of your calories will keep you focused on your meal plan.

Eating out at restaurants is another part of your meal plan. Based on your schedule you may need to eat out several times a week. Here are some tips on how to stick to your meal plan when eating out.

Make a list of the restaurants you frequent. Narrow the list based on the restaurants that offer healthy low calorie options. There are several restaurants that now have a specific menu for people who are counting calories. Once you have the list narrowed down, only eat at the restaurants on your list. When friends invite you out to eat, let them know up front that there are only certain restaurants you frequent.

Never accept free appetizers such as bread or chips and salsa. This will become easier. You will create a habit that becomes routine.

Study the menu carefully and use your smartphone to get the calorie counts before you make your selection.

Take your time and enjoy your meal. Consider it a treat to be dining out.

For families, changing eating habits can be difficult and kids love junk food. Having a healthier eating environment can create lifelong nutritious eating habits.

If your family is all-in on creating a healthy eating environment, then make a clean slate. Get the foods you don't need out of your house. If you aren't looking at the foods you crave you are less likely to eat them. Stock your fridge and pantry with nutritious choices. It will allow you and your family to become accustomed to eating healthy food and creating a lifestyle change.

Educate your family on the benefits of healthy eating. Keep the information basic and simple. This makes it easier for children to understand the advantages of changing their diet. If you need help in talking to your children about healthy eating, search the web. There are all kinds of sources for you to use to educate your children on the benefits of healthy eating.

If putting the entire family on a healthier eating plan is not something that can be done overnight, try limiting the junk food and keep it stored in a container that is not visibly seen.

Make slow gradual food changes for the family.
Slowly incorporating more healthy food over time can
make the transitions easier for the entire family.

I have attached a sample meal plan at the end of this book.
Feel free to use to create your own meal plan.

Staying Focused On Your Exercise Plan

Exercise is a must have component of any weight loss program. You consume calories and you will need to burn them off. Here are some tips to help you with the exercise portion of your program.

Schedule your workouts. On the days you plan to work out, make them a part of your daily routine.

Schedule things around your workout. Your workout time is for you. Do your best to not let other things interfere.

Incorporate cardio and strength training into every workout. If you want to work out an hour a day four days a week, split the time between 30 minutes' cardio and 30 minutes' strength training.

Find exercises you enjoy. This makes your workout fun and more likely to continue it long term. If strength training isn't your thing, that is ok. If you like to bike then bike. If aerobics is your thing, then go for it. The more enjoyable your workouts are the happier you will be. Exercise releases endorphins so take advantage and have fun.

Push through the tough days. There are going to be days where you will struggle. Keep your head up and push through your obstacles. Don't let barriers stand in your way.

Don't make excuses to miss your workout. One excuse leads to more excuses, and before you realize it you have quit exercising altogether.

Add music to your work out. Build a workout playlist and listen to it while you are exercising. This helps keep you focused on your workout and from getting distracted from outside forces.

Set goals. Reaching milestones will only motivate you to go further.

Get a workout buddy. Having a workout partner will help keep you accountable to your gym schedule and reaching fitness goals.

Get in your zone. Athletes do this before a sporting event and so can you. Before you begin your workout mentally prepare yourself for it. Think about your exercise routine and give yourself a pep talk to pump yourself up. There are all kinds of motivational quotes you can find online to help you boost your confidence before you work out.

Don't be intimidated by the gym. You are there for the same reason as everyone else; to exercise. People may judge you but so be it. That is on them not you. Keep your focus on you and your workout. Music can help you to stay focused and block out everything else.

Get the family involved. Try exercising as a family. Break out some of the dance games available on electronic gaming devices. Try outdoor activities, such as basketball, volleyball, soccer, kickball, bike riding, or walking.

How To Stay Mentally Motivated

Mental Motivation is the most important aspect to any weight loss program. Our brains are one of the most powerful tools we have within us. We make the decision to eat right and exercise just as we choose to eat unhealthy and not work out. Keeping mental focus in the forefront of your weight loss journey will motivate you to continually move forward

Find motivational quotes that reflect your weight loss journey and touch you in a personal way. Creating a personal connection with a motivational quote adds value and you are more likely to remain focused on your goals.

Set daily reminders on your phone and/or email calendar throughout your day to keep you focused on your goals. Use motivational quotes covering different aspects of your journey. My work schedule was 8 a.m. to 5 p.m. Driving to work was stressful, so I made sure to have a motivational quote pop up in my reminders at 8 a.m. This helped me start my day on a positive note. I also had a reminder set for around lunch-time to encourage me to make healthy choices if I ate out. Towards the end of the day I had another reminder set so that I would be motivated to work out after I left work for the day.

Create a vision board. A vision board is a board you create using poster board. You can write, draw or glue anything you want on this board. Some examples are motivational quotes, magazine, or newspaper clippings. You can write out specific goals you want to achieve along your journey. There are a ton of examples on the internet. Do a search and get creative with your board. Also, once it is complete place the board somewhere you will see it each day. Take a picture of it and use it as your background on your phone or print the picture and place in a small frame on your desk or somewhere in your home.

Keep a journal. Document your journey and when you are having a bad day, write about it. This can help you work on the struggles you face by pinpointing specific issues that affect your weight loss quest.

Build a support team for yourself. Reach out to your friends, family, and co-workers. Ask them to support you along your journey. Try to choose individuals that will rally to your cause. Also, assign tasks to your team. A great example is to have one person be your support for fitness, one for your diet/meal plan and one for mental motivation. Select individuals who are strong suited for the task.

Don't go at it alone. If you have someone who has similar goals reach out to them and hopefully the two of you can do this together.

I hope these tips will help you along your journey. The most important piece of advice I can give you is to make this journey your own. Personalize it to your lifestyle and make sure your plan follows suit. Your plan should be modifiable to your likes and dislikes. This will go a long way with your journey.

If you have experienced a long and/or tough struggle with weight loss, I want you to know that you are not alone. You can do this and I can help you. I started my business because I am passionate about helping others succeed in their journey.

A Weigh To Lose Weight Loss Center

A Weigh To Lose is a company built on a "No Pills, No Potions, No Products" platform. The company provides meal plans, exercise plans, and coaching. The great thing about our programs is that they can be done in our office or online. If you don't live near Conway, Arkansas, that is ok. I can still help you. The programs can be done virtually. Coaching is done through Skype.

The best thing about the programs is that your meal plans and workouts are delivered through an app that you can access on your smartphone or tablet. Your program goes with you. You will absolutely love the workouts. They come with instructional videos that show you the proper form and technique. It's like having a personal trainer at your fingertips

Each program comes with coaching. My virtual clients love Skype coaching because they can do it at their work while on a break or at home while relaxing in their pajamas. Coaching through Skype also makes them more comfortable to openly express their feelings. The reason for this is clients are usually Skyping from the comfort of their own home. Talking about sensitive subjects in a safe environment gives the client the opportunity to be more open with their feelings.

In coaching, we first go over your program and discuss any questions, concerns, or comments you may have. The second half of the coaching is focused on mental motivation. We may discuss issues that affect you focus or do a mental motivational exercise during your session.

I believe that getting coaching through someone that knows and understands your struggle is so important. We can relate to each other on a personal level. Individuals that use my program are not just clients; they are also friends. I care about their journey and I want them to achieve their goals.

For those that live locally we are also incorporating small group strength classes. These classes are not only fun they are effective. Having a small group keeps us all focused on our fitness goals. Another great thing about the groups is that they are very affordable. Anyone on a budget can enjoy these classes.

I hope you can take this book and apply what you have read to your weight loss journey. If nothing else, I hope it invigorates you to continue to strive for your goals.

As I said in the beginning of this book, I've never completed a diet or weight loss program because this is a journey as well as a lifestyle change. It is not only ever evolving, but it will always be a part of my life personally and professionally.

If you are interested in becoming an in-office or virtual client, please contact me. Virtual and in-office consultations are free. You can reach me several different ways listed below.

Email: aweightolose@gmail.com

Website: www.aweightolose.com

Facebook: www.facebook.com/aweightolose

Phone: 501-327-2123

Tell your friends about this book by sharing this link below:

www.kimlmcpherson.com

Sample Meal Plan

This sample meal plan can be used to help you build your own meal plan as well give you an idea how we design meal plans at A Weigh To Lose.

Breakfast

½ c. oatmeal

¼ c. fresh fruit

1 egg poached or scrambled

Mid Morning or Mid Afternoon Snack

1 cup of Greek yogurt or

1 piece of fruit (apple, banana, orange, peach etc.) or

½ c veggies sticks with light ranch dressing

Lunch

4-6 oz. of grilled chicken

2 leaves of romaine lettuce

2 slices tomato

2 tbs. shredded carrot

2 tbs. light dressing

1 tbs shredded parmesan cheese

1 piece of fruit (apple, banana, orange, peach etc.)

Mid Afternoon Snack or After Dinner Snack

1 cup Greek yogurt or

1 protein bar or

1 serving of light ice cream or frozen yogurt

Dinner

4-6 oz. lean hamburger patty or sirloin steak

1 c. mixed vegetables (steamed, broiled, boiled, etc.)

1 small baked or roasted potato

1 small dinner salad with 2 tbs. with light dressing.

About The Author

I was born and raised in Arkansas. I have a degree in Finance and I am a Certified Lifestyles & Weight Management Specialist. I have always wanted to be an entrepreneur and author. I finally decided to take the plunge and do both. I have started my own weight loss center in Conway, Arkansas and became an author.

I love the fact that my business is done nationwide. It gives me the opportunity to meet new and exciting people every day. I want the business to grow nationally and franchise into centers across the United States.

Being an author is a dream come true. I not only write self-help books, I also write romance novels. Having the ability to share ideas with others is a great outlet for me.

I love the person I am becoming as well as what I do. Having a career I love and helping others is a dream come true for me. I also enjoy reading, spending time with my family, and cooking. I plan writing more books on weight loss but my next project is a cookbook.

If you would like to receive updates on upcoming projects and books email me at the address below:

Email: aweightolose@gmail.com